Mediterranean Every Day

Simple Weeknight Recipes from the World's Healthiest Cuisine

By Enola Gekko

Sommario

INTRODUCTION

The Mediterranean Diet constitutes a set of knowledge and traditions ranging from landscape to table, including crops, harvesting, fishing, conservation, processing, preparation, and consumption of food.

It is characterized by a nutritional model that has remained constant in time and places, being mainly made up of: olive oil, cereals, fresh and dried fruits, vegetables, a moderate amount of fish, dairy products, meat, many seasonings, and spices, entirely accompanied by wine. It is a model of a sustainable diet, as it contributes to preserve: quality, food, and nutritional safety and at the same time promotes the management of environmental and territorial resources.

Mediterranean diet is a specific diet by removing processed foods and high in saturated fats. It's not necessarily about losing weight, but rather a healthy lifestyle choice. It is about ingesting traditional ingredients consumed by those who have lived in the Mediterranean basin for a long time. This is a diet rich in fruits, vegetables, and fish. Cooking with olive oil is a fundamental ingredient and is an ideal replacement for saturated fats. Studies show that the people who live in these regions live longer and better lives.

CHAPTER 1: BREAKFAST RECIPES

Cooked Beef Mushroom Egg

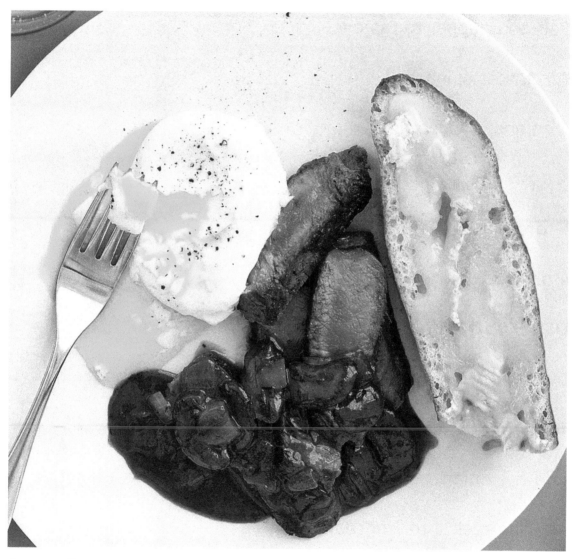

Servings: 2

Preparation time: 15 minutes

INGREDIENTS

- ¼ cup cooked beef, diced

- 6 eggs

- 4 mushrooms, diced

- Salt and pepper to taste

- 12 ounces spinach

- 2 onions, chopped

- A dash of onion powder

- ¼ green bell pepper, chopped

- A dash of garlic powder

DIRECTIONS

In a skillet, toss the beef for 3 minutes or until crispy.

Take off the heat and add to a plate.

Add the onion, bell pepper, and mushroom to the skillet.

Add the rest of the ingredients.

Toss for about 4 minutes.

Return the beef to the skillet and toss for another minute.

Serve hot

NUTRITION Calories 213, Fat 15.7g, Carbs 3.4g, Protein 14.5g

Tropical Almond Pancakes

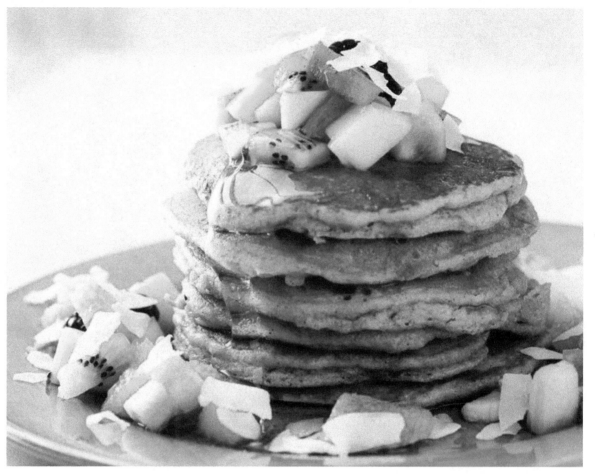

Servings: 8

Preparation time: 15 minutes

INGREDIENTS

- 2 cups creamy milk

- 3 ½ cups almond flour

- 1 tsp baking soda

- ½ tsp salt

- 1 tsp allspice

- 2 tbsp vanilla

- 1 tsp cinnamon

- 1 tsp baking powder

- ½ cup club soda

DIRECTIONS

1. Preheat the Airfryer at 290F and grease the cooking basket of the air fryer.

2. Whisk together salt, almond flour, baking soda, allspice, and cinnamon in a large bowl.

3. Mix together the vanilla, baking powder, and club soda and add to the flour mixture.

4. Stir the mixture thoroughly and pour the mixture into the cooking basket.

5. Cook for about 10 minutes and dish out on a serving platter.

NUTRITION Calories 324, Fat 24.5g, Carbs 12.8g, Protein 11.5g, Sugar 1.6g, Sodium 342mg

Spiced Breakfast Casserole

Servings: 6

Preparation time: 55 mins

INGREDIENTS

12 to 16 ounces smoked andouille sausage (thinly sliced)

1/2 cup chopped onion

1/2 cup chopped red or green bell pepper

6 large eggs

1 1/2 cups milk

1 teaspoon Creole or Cajun seasoning blend

1/4 teaspoon black pepper

1 tablespoon fresh chopped parsley (optional)

4 slices bread torn into 1-inch pieces (or use 2 large croissants, sliced sandwich-style and torn)

2 medium tomatoes (diced)

2 cups shredded Cheddar cheese

Salt and pepper

DIRECTIONS

1. Heat oven to 350 F/180 C/Gas 4.

2. Butter a shallow 2-quart baking dish. In a large skillet, cook sliced sausage with the onion and bell pepper until vegetables are translucent.

3. Whisk eggs with milk in a bowl with the Creole seasoning, pepper, and parsley, if using; set aside. Arrange the torn bread pieces over the bottom of the buttered baking dish. Sprinkle with the sausage mixture and the diced tomatoes.

4. Top with Cheddar cheese, then pour the egg mixture evenly over the top. Sprinkle with salt and pepper. Bake the casserole for 35 to 40 minutes, or until it is puffy and lightly browned.

NUTRITION Calories 604, Fat 46g, Carbs 13g, Protein 34g

Paleo Almond Banana Pancakes

Servings: 2

Preparation time: 10 mins

INGREDIENTS

- 1 cup almond flour

- 3 tablespoons tapioca flour

- 1.5 teaspoons baking powder

- pinch of kosher salt

- 1/4 cup unsweetened almond milk

- 1 Happy Egg Free Range egg

- 1 tablespoon maple syrup

- 1 teaspoon vanilla extract

- 1 banana, 1/3 mashed + 1/2 chopped

DIRECTIONS

In a large bowl, combine almond flour, tapioca flour, baking powder, and salt. Gently whisk all ingredients together with a fork.

In the same bowl, combine almond milk, one Happy Egg Free Range egg, maple syrup, banana, and vanilla extract. Gently stir until everything has come together. Heat a medium non-stick skillet over medium heat and coat with butter or coconut oil. Scoop 1/4 cup pancake batter and pour into the pan to form a small to medium-sized pancake. Cook for 2-3 minutes or until the edges begin to puff and the bottom is golden brown. Flip and cook for another two minutes or until cooked through. Repeat until you have worked through all the batter. Serve + enjoy!

Notes: If you don't have tapioca flour, you can sub in arrowroot or cornstarch! If you are not gluten-free, you can also sub wheat flour for the tapioca.

NUTRITION Serving: 4 pancakes Calories 480, Carbohydrates 44g, Protein 15g, Fat 30g, Saturated Fat 3g, Cholesterol 82mg, Sodium 76mg, Potassium 567mg, Fiber 7g, Sugar 16g, Calcium 308mg, Iron 3mg

Quinoa Fruit Salad

Servings: 4

Preparation time: 25 mins

INGREDIENTS

For the Quinoa:

- 1 cup quinoa

- 2 cups water

- Pinch of salt

- 3 tablespoons honey

For the Honey Lime Dressing:

- Juice of 1 large lime

- 2 tablespoons finely chopped fresh mint

For the fruit:

- 1 1/2 cups blueberries

- 1 1/2 cups sliced strawberries

- 1 1/2 cups chopped mango Extra chopped mint for garnish-optional

DIRECTIONS

1. Using a strainer, rinse the quinoa under cold water. Add quinoa, water, and salt to a medium saucepan and bring to a boil over medium heat. Boil for 5 minutes.

2. Turn the heat to low and simmer for about 15 minutes or until water is absorbed. Remove from heat and fluff with a fork. Let quinoa cool to room temperature.

3. To make the Honey Lime Dressing: In a medium bowl, whisk the lime juice, honey, and mint together until combined. In a large bowl, combine quinoa, blueberries, strawberries, and mango. Pour honey lime dressing over the fruit salad and mix until well combined.

4. Garnish with additional mint, if desired. Serve at room temperature or chilled.

5. Note: Use your favorite fruit in this salad. Blackberries, peaches, kiwi, raspberries, pineapple, grapes, etc., are great options!

NUTRITION Calories 308,1, Fat 18.2g, Saturated Fat 2.2g, Cholesterol 0mg, Sodium 10mg, Total Carbohydrate 34.1g, Dietary Fiber 4.5g, Sugars 15.2g, Protein 4.4g

Baked Avocado Eggs

Servings: 4

Preparation time: 30 mins

INGREDIENTS

- 3 avocados, halved and seeded

- 6 large eggs

- Kosher salt and freshly ground black pepper to taste

- 2 tablespoons chopped fresh chives

DIRECTIONS

1. Preheat oven to 400°F (200°C). Slice the avocados in half and remove the pits. Place the avocado halves on a baking sheet and scoop out some of the flesh to make a bigger hole. Crack one egg into each hole and season with salt and pepper. Top with toppings of choice and bake for 15 minutes or until yolk reaches desired consistency. Sprinkle with fresh herbs, as desired. Enjoy!

NUTRITION: Calories 249, Fat 19g, Carbs 9g, Fiber 5g, Sugar 0g, Protein 11g

Keto Breakfast Pizza

Servings: 6

Preparation time: 30 mins

INGREDIENTS

- 2 tablespoons coconut flour

- 2 cups cauliflower, grated

- ½ teaspoon salt

- 1 tablespoon psyllium husk powder

- 4 eggs

Toppings:

- Avocado

- Smoked Salmon

- Herbs

- Olive oil

- Spinach

DIRECTIONS

1. Preheat the oven to 360 degrees F and grease a pizza tray.

2. Mix together all ingredients in a bowl, except toppings, and keep aside.

3. Pour the pizza dough onto the pan and mold it into an even pizza crust using your hands.

4. Top the pizza with toppings and transfer in the oven.

5. Bake for about 15 minutes until golden brown and remove from the oven to serve.

   NUTRITION Calories 454, Carbs 16g, Fat 31g, Protein 22g, Sodium 1325mg, Sugar 4.4g

Pumpkin Pancakes

Servings: 8

Preparation time: 20 minutes

INGREDIENTS

- 2 squares puff pastry

- 6 tbsp pumpkin filling

- 2 small eggs, beaten

- ¼ tsp cinnamon

DIRECTIONS

Preheat the Airfryer to 360 F and roll out a square of puff pastry.

Layer it with pumpkin pie filling, leaving about 1/4 -inch space around the edges.

Cut it up into equal sized square pieces and cover the gaps with beaten egg.

Arrange the squares into a baking dish and cook for about 12 minutes.

Sprinkle some cinnamon and serve

NUTRITION Calories 51, Carbs 5g, Fat 2.5g, Protein 2.4g, Sugar 0.5g

Baked Eggs with Cheddar and Beef

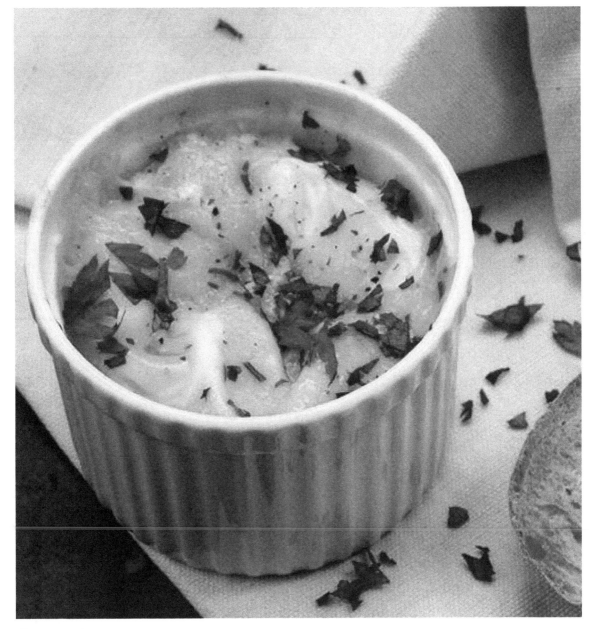

Servings: 2

Preparation time: 10 minutes

INGREDIENTS

3 oz ground beef, cooked

2 organic eggs

2 oz shredded cheddar cheese

1 tbsp olive oil

DIRECTION

Switch on the oven, then set its temperature to 390F and let it preheat.

Meanwhile, take a baking dish, grease it with oil, add spread cooked beef in the bottom, then make two holes in it and crack an organic egg into each hole.

Sprinkle cheese on top of beef and eggs and bake for 20 minutes until beef has cooked and eggs have set.

When done, let baked eggs cool for 5 minutes and then serve straight away.

For meal prepping, wrap baked eggs in foil and refrigerate for up to two days.

When ready to eat, reheat baked eggs in the microwave and then serve.

NUTRITION: Calories 512, Total Fat 32.8g, Total Carbs 1.4g, Protein 51g, Sugar 1g, Sodium 531mg

Paleo Chocolate Banana Bread

Servings: 10

Preparation time: 50 minutes

INGREDIENTS

¼ cup dark chocolate, chopped

½ cup almond butter

½ cup coconut flour, sifted

½ teaspoon cinnamon powder

1 teaspoon baking soda

1 teaspoon vanilla extract

4 bananas, mashed

4 eggs

4 tablespoon coconut oil, melted

A pinch of salt

DIRECTIONS

1. Preheat the oven to 350F.

2. Grease an 8" x 8" square pan and set it aside.

3. In a large bowl, mix together the eggs, banana, vanilla extract, almond butter, and coconut oil. Mix well until well combined.

4. Add the cinnamon powder, coconut flour, baking powder, baking soda, and salt to the wet ingredients. Fold until well combined. Add in the chopped chocolates, then fold the batter again.

5. Pour the batter into the greased pan. Spread evenly.

6. Bake in the oven for about 50 minutes or until a toothpick inserted in the center comes out clean.

7. Remove from the hot oven and cool on a wire rack for an hour.

NUTRITION Calories: 150.3: Carbs: 13.9g; Protein: 3.2g; Fat: 9.1g

Baked Eggs and Asparagus with Parmesan

Servings: 2

Preparation time: 30 mins

INGREDIENTS

- 4 eggs

- 8 thick asparagus spears, cut into bite-sized pieces

- 2 teaspoons olive oil

- 2 tablespoons Parmesan cheese

- Salt and black pepper to taste

DIRECTIONS

Preheat the oven to 400 degrees F and grease two gratin dishes with olive oil.

Put half the asparagus into each gratin dish and place in the oven.

Roast for about 10 minutes and dish out the gratin dishes.

Baked Eggs and Asparagus with Parmesan

Crack eggs over the asparagus and transfer into the oven.

Bake for about 5 minutes and dish out the dishes.

Sprinkle with Parmesan cheese and put the dishes back in the oven.

Bake for another 3 minutes and dish out to serve hot.

NUTRITION: Calories: 336 Carbs: 13.7g Fat: 19.4g Protein: 28.1g Sodium: 2103mg Sugar: 4.7g

Zucchini and Quinoa Pan

Servings: 4

Preparation time: 20 Minutes

INGREDIENTS

1 tablespoon olive oil

2 garlic cloves, minced

1 cup quinoa

1 zucchini, roughly cubed

2 tablespoons basil, chopped

¼ cup green olives, pitted and chopped

1 tomato, cubed

½ cup feta cheese, crumbled

2 cups water

1 cup canned garbanzo beans, drained and rinsed

A pinch of salt and black pepper

DIRECTION

Heat up a pan with the oil over medium-high heat, add the garlic and quinoa and brown for 3 minutes.

Add the water, zucchinis, salt, and pepper, toss, bring to a simmer, and cook for 15 minutes.

Add the rest of the ingredients, toss, divide everything between plates and serve for breakfast.

NUTRITION Calories 310, Fat 11g, Fiber 6g, Carbs 42g, Protein 11g

Peas Omelet

Servings: 6

Preparation time: 20 minutes

INGREDIENTS

- 4 oz green peas

- ¼ cup corn kernels

- 6 eggs, beaten

- ¼ cup heavy cream

- ½ teaspoon of sea salt

- 1 red bell pepper, chopped

- 1 teaspoon butter

- ½ teaspoon paprika

DIRECTION

1. Toss butter in the skillet and melt it.

2. Add green peas, bell pepper, and corn kernels. Start to roast the vegetables over medium heat.

3. Meanwhile, in the mixing bowl, whisk together eggs, heavy cream, sea salt, and paprika.

4. Pour the mixture over the roasted vegetables and stir well immediately.

5. Close the lid and cook the omelet over medium-low heat for 15 minutes or until it is solid.

6. Transfer the cooked omelet to the big plate and cut it into servings.

NUTRITION Calories 113, Fat 7.1g, Fiber 1.5g, Carbs 6g, Protein 7.1g

Breakfast Egg-Artichoke Casserole

Servings: 8

Preparation time: 35 minutes

INGREDIENTS

16 large eggs

14 ounce can artichoke hearts, drained

10-ounce box frozen chopped spinach, thawed and drained well

1 cup shredded white cheddar

1 garlic clove, minced

1 teaspoon salt

½ cup parmesan cheese

½ cup ricotta cheese

½ teaspoon dried thyme

½ teaspoon crushed red pepper

¼ cup milk

¼p shaved onion

DIRECTIONS

Lightly grease a 9x13-inch baking dish with cooking spray and preheat the oven to 350F.

In a large mixing bowl, add eggs and milk. Mix thoroughly.

With a paper towel, squeeze out the excess moisture from the spinach leaves and add to the bowl of eggs.

Into small pieces, break the artichoke hearts and separate the leaves. Add to the bowl of eggs.

Except for the ricotta cheese, add the remaining ingredients in the bowl of eggs and mix thoroughly.

Pour egg mixture into the prepared dish.

Evenly add dollops of ricotta cheese on top of the eggs and then pop in the oven.

Bake until eggs are set and don't jiggle when shook, about 35 minutes.

Remove from the oven and evenly divide into suggested servings. Enjoy.

NUTRITION Calories : 302; Protein: 22.6g; Carbs: 10.8g; Fat: 18.7g

Protein-Packed Blender Pancakes

Servings: 1

Preparation time: 15 minutes

INGREDIENTS

2 organic eggs

1 scoop protein powder

Salt to taste

¼ tsp cinnamon

2 oz cream cheese, softened

1 tsp unsalted butter

INSTRUCTIONS

1. Crack the eggs in a blender, add remaining ingredients except for butter, and pulse for 2 minutes until well combined and blended.

2. Take a skillet pan, place it over medium heat, add butter and when it melts, pour in prepared batter, spread it evenly, and cook for 4 to 5 minutes per side until cooked through and golden brown.

3. Serve straight away.

NUTRITION Calories 450, Total Fat 29g, Total Carbs 4g, Protein 41g

Avocado Egg Scramble

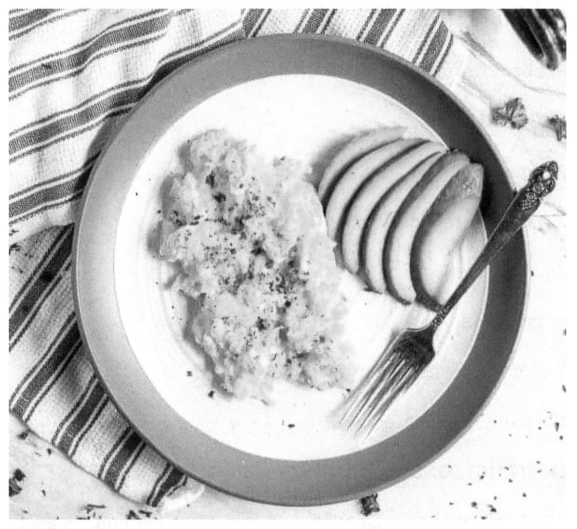

Servings: 4

Preparation time: 25 minutes

INGREDIENTS

4 eggs, beaten

1 white onion, diced

1 tablespoon avocado oil

1 avocado, finely chopped

½ teaspoon chili flakes

1 oz Cheddar cheese, shredded

½ teaspoon salt

1 tablespoon fresh parsley

DIRECTIONS

1. Pour avocado oil into the skillet and bring it to a boil.

2. Then add diced onion and roast it until it is light brown.

3. Meanwhile, mix up together chili flakes, beaten eggs, and salt

4. Pour the egg mixture over the cooked onion and cook the mixture for 1 minute over medium heat.

5. After this, scramble the eggs well with the help of the fork or spatula. Cook the eggs until they are solid but soft.

6. After this, add chopped avocado and shredded cheese.

7. Stir well and transfer to serving plates.

8. Sprinkle the meal with fresh parsley.

NUTRITION Calories 236, Fat 20.1g, Fiber 4g, Carbs 7.4g, Protein 8.6g

Avocado and Eggs Breakfast Tacos

Servings: 2

Preparation time: 23 minutes

INGREDIENTS

4 organic eggs

1 tbsp unsalted butter

2 low-carb tortillas

2 tbsp mayonnaise

4 sprigs of cilantro

½ of an avocado, sliced

Salt and freshly cracked black pepper to taste

1 tbsp Tabasco sauce

INSTRUCTIONS

Take a bowl, crack eggs in it and whisk well until smooth.

Take a skillet pan, place it over medium heat, add butter and when it melts, pour in eggs, spread them evenly in the pan, and cook for 4 to 5 minutes until done.

When done, transfer eggs to a plate and set aside until required.

Add tortillas into the pan, cook for 2 to 3 minutes per side until warm through, and then transfer them onto a plate.

Assemble tacos and for this, spread mayonnaise on the side of each tortilla, then distribute cooked eggs and top with cilantro and sliced avocado.

Season with salt and black pepper, drizzle with tabasco sauce, and roll up the tortillas.

Serve straight away or store in the refrigerator for two days until ready to eat.

NUTRITION Calories 289, Total Fat 27g, Total Carbs 6g, Protein 7g

Low Carb Green Smoothie

Servings: 2

Preparation time: 15 minutes

INGREDIENTS

- 1/ 3 cup romaine lettuce

- 1/3 tablespoon fresh ginger, peeled and chopped

- 1 ½ cups filtered water

- 1/8 cup fresh pineapple, chopped

- ¾ tablespoon fresh parsley

- 1/3 raw cucumber, peeled and sliced

- ¼ Hass avocado

- ¼ cup kiwi fruit, peeled and chopped

- 1/3 tablespoon Swerve

DIRECTION

1. Put all the ingredients in a blender and blend until smooth.

2. Pour into 2 serving glasses and serve chilled.

   NUTRITION Calories: 108, Carbs: 7.8g, Fat: 8.9g, Protein: 1.6g, Sodium: 4 mg, Sugar: 2.2g

Vanilla Oats

Servings: 4

Preparation time: 10 Minutes

INGREDIENTS

- ½ cup rolled oats

- 1 cup milk

- 1 teaspoon vanilla extract

- 1 teaspoon ground cinnamon

- 2 teaspoon honey

- 2 tablespoons Plain yogurt

- 1 teaspoon butter

DIRECTION

Pour milk into the saucepan and bring it to a boil.

Add rolled oats and stir well.

Close the lid and simmer the oats for 5 minutes over medium heat. The cooked oats will absorb all milk.

Then add butter and stir the oats well.

In the separated bowl, whisk together Plain yogurt with honey, cinnamon, and vanilla extract.

Transfer the cooked oats to the serving bowls.

Top the oats with the yogurt mixture in the shape of the wheel.

NUTRITION Calories 243, Fat 20.2, Fiber 1g, Carbs 2.8g, Protein 13.3g

Orzo and Veggie Bowls

Servings: 4

Preparation time: 0 minutes

INGREDIENTS

- 2 and ½ cups whole-wheat orzo, cooked

- 14 ounces canned cannellini beans, drained and rinsed

- 1 yellow bell pepper, cubed

- 1 green bell pepper, cubed

- A pinch of salt and black pepper

- 3 tomatoes, cubed

- 1 red onion, chopped

- 1 cup mint, chopped

- 2 cups feta cheese, crumbled

- 2 tablespoons olive oil

- ¼ cup lemon juice

- 1 tablespoon lemon zest, grated

- 1 cucumber, cubed

- 1 and ¼ cup kalamata olives, pitted and sliced

- 3 garlic cloves, minced

DIRECTIONS

In a salad bowl, combine the orzo with the beans, bell peppers, and the rest of the ingredients, toss, divide the mix between plates and serve for breakfast.

NUTRITION Calories 411, Fat 17g, Fiber 13g, Carbs 51g, Protein 14g

Spiced Chickpeas Bowls

Servings: 4

Preparation time: 30 minutes

INGREDIENTS

15 ounces canned chickpeas, drained and rinsed

¼ teaspoon cardamom, ground

½ teaspoon cinnamon powder

1 and ½ teaspoons turmeric powder

1 teaspoon coriander, ground

1 tablespoon olive oil

A pinch of salt and black pepper

¾ cup Greek yogurt

½ cup green olives, pitted and halved

½ cup cherry tomatoes, halved

1 cucumber, sliced

DIRECTIONS

2. Spread the chickpeas on a lined baking sheet, add the cardamom, cinnamon, turmeric, coriander, oil, salt, and pepper, toss and bake at 375 degrees F for 30 minutes.

3. In a bowl, combine the roasted chickpeas with the rest of the ingredients, toss and serve for breakfast.

   NUTRITION Calories 519, Fat 34.5g, Fiber 13.3g, Carbs 49.8g, Protein 12g

Mediterranean Egg Feta Scramble

Servings: 4

Preparation time: 15 minutes

INGREDIENTS

- 6 eggs

- ¾ cup crumbled feta cheese

- 2 tablespoons green onions, minced

- 2 tablespoons red peppers, roasted, diced

- ¼ teaspoon kosher salt

- ¼ teaspoon garlic powder

- ¼ cup Greek yogurt

- ½ teaspoon dry oregano

- ½ teaspoon dry basil

- 1 teaspoon olive oil

- A few cracks freshly ground black pepper

- Warm whole-wheat tortillas, optional

DIRECTIONS

1. Preheat a skillet over medium heat.

2. In a bowl, whisk the eggs, sour cream, basil, oregano, garlic powder, salt, and pepper. Gently add the feta.

3. When the skillet is hot, add the olive oil and then the egg mixture; allow the egg mix to set, then scrape the bottom of the pan to let the uncooked egg cook. Stir in the red peppers and the green onions.

4. Continue cooking until the egg mixture is cooked to your preferred doneness. Serve immediately.

5. If desired, sprinkle with extra feta and then wrap the scrambled eggs in tortillas.

NUTRITION Calories 260, Fat 16g, Chol 350mg, Sodium 750mg, Pot. 190mg, Carb. 12g, Sugar 2g, Protein 16g

Fig with Ricotta Oatmeal

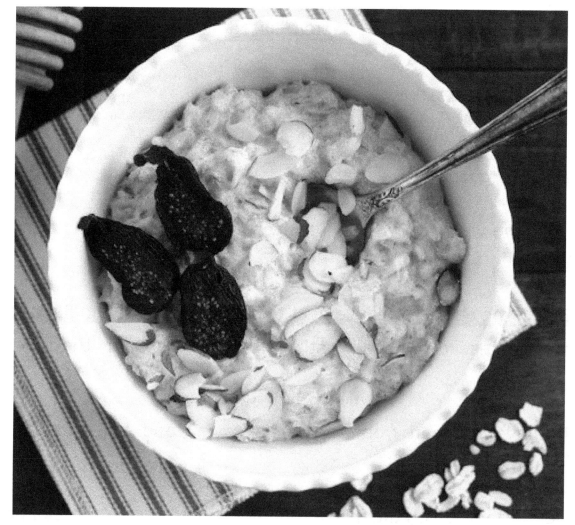

Servings: 1

Preparation time: 5 minutes

INGREDIENTS

2 teaspoons honey

2 tablespoons ricotta cheese, part-skin

2 tablespoons dried figs, chopped

½ cup old-fashioned rolled oats

1 tablespoon almonds, toasted, sliced

1 cup water

Pinch of salt

DIRECTIONS

1. Pour the water into a small saucepan and add the salt; bring to a boil.

2. Stir in the oats and reduce heat to medium. Cook the oats for about 5 minutes, occasionally stirring, until most of the water is absorbed.

3. Remove the pan from the heat, cover, and let stand for 2-3 minutes.

4. Serve topped with the figs, almonds, ricotta, and a drizzle of honey.

NUTRITION Calories 315, Fat 8g, Chol. 10mg, Sodium 194mg, Pot. 359mg, Fiber 7g, Protein 10g

Breakfast Tostadas

Servings: 6

Preparation time: 6 Minutes

INGREDIENTS

- ½ white onion, diced

- 1 tomato, chopped

- 1 cucumber, chopped

- 1 tablespoon fresh cilantro, chopped

- ½ jalapeno pepper, chopped

- 1 tablespoon lime juice

- 6 corn tortillas

- 1 tablespoon canola oil

- 2 oz Cheddar cheese, shredded

- ½ cup white beans, canned, drained

- 6 eggs

- ½ teaspoon butter

- ½ teaspoon Sea salt

DIRECTIONS

1. Make Pico de Gallo: in the salad bowl, combine together diced white onion, tomato, cucumber, fresh cilantro, and jalapeno pepper.

2. Then add lime juice and a ½ tablespoon of canola oil. Mix up the mixture well. Pico de Gallo is cooked.

3. Then, preheat the oven to 390F.

4. Line the tray with baking paper.

5. Arrange the corn tortillas on the baking paper and brush with canola oil from both sides.

6. Bake the tortillas for 10 minutes or until they start to be crunchy.

7. Chill the cooked crunchy tortillas well.

8. Meanwhile, toss the butter in the skillet.

9. Crack the eggs in the melted butter and sprinkle them with sea salt.

10. Fry the eggs until the egg whites become white (cooked). Approximately for 3-5 minutes over medium heat.

11. After this, mash the beans until you get a puree texture.

12. Spread the bean puree on the corn tortillas.

13. Add fried eggs.

14.   Then top the eggs with Pico de Gallo and shredded Cheddar cheese.

NUTRITION Calories 246, Fat 11.1g, Fiber 4.7g, Carbs 24.5g, Protein 13.7g

Raspberry Pudding

Servings: 2

Preparation time: 30 minutes

INGREDIENTS

½ cup raspberries

2 teaspoons maple syrup

1 ½ cup Plain yogurt

¼ teaspoon ground cardamom

1/3 cup Chia seeds, dried

DIRECTIONS

Mix up together Plain yogurt with maple syrup and ground cardamom.

Add Chia seeds. Stir it gently.

Put the yogurt in the serving glasses and top with the raspberries.

Refrigerate the breakfast for at least 3 minutes or overnight.

NUTRITION Calories 303, Fat 11.2g, Fiber 11.8g, Carbs 33.2g, Protein 15.5g

Walnuts Yogurt Mix

Servings: 6

Preparation time: 0 Minutes

INGREDIENTS

- 2 and ½ cups Greek yogurt

- 1 and ½ cups walnuts, chopped

- 1 teaspoon vanilla extract

- ¾ cup honey

- 2 teaspoons cinnamon powder

DIRECTIONS

In a bowl, combine the yogurt with the walnuts and the rest of the ingredients, toss, divide into smaller bowls and keep in the fridge for 10 minutes before serving for breakfast.

NUTRITION Calories 388, Fat 24.6g, Fiber 2.9g, Carbs 39.1g, Protein 10.2g

Mushroom Egg Casserole

Servings: 3

Preparation time: 25 minutes

INGREDIENTS

½ cup mushrooms, chopped

½ yellow onion, diced

4 eggs, beaten

1 tablespoon coconut flakes

½ teaspoon chili pepper

1 oz Cheddar cheese, shredded

1 teaspoon canola oil

DIRECTIONS

1. Pour canola oil in the skillet and preheat well.

2. Add mushrooms and onion and roast for 5-8 minutes or until the vegetables are light brown.

3. Transfer the cooked vegetables to the casserole mold.

4. Add coconut flakes, chili pepper, and Cheddar cheese.

5. Then add eggs and stir well.

6. Bake the casserole for 15 minutes at 360F.

NUTRITION Calories 152, Fat 11.1, Fiber 0.7, Carbs 3g, Protein 10.4g

Bacon Veggies Combo

Servings: 2

Preparation time: 35 minutes

INGREDIENTS

½ green bell pepper, seeded and chopped

2 bacon slices

¼ cup Parmesan Cheese

½ tablespoon mayonnaise

1 scallion, chopped

DIRECTIONS

1. Preheat the oven to 375 degrees F and grease a baking dish.

2. Place bacon slices on the baking dish and top with mayonnaise, bell peppers, scallions, and Parmesan Cheese.

3. Transfer in the oven and bake for about 25 minutes.

4. Dish out to serve immediately or refrigerate for about a day, wrapped in a plastic sheet for meal prepping.

NUTRITION Calories 197, Fat 13.8g, Carbohydrates 4.7g, Protein 14.3g, Sugar 1.9g, Sodium 662mg

Brown Rice Salad

Servings: 4

Preparation time: 0 Minutes

INGREDIENTS

9 ounces brown rice, cooked

7 cups baby arugula

15 ounces canned garbanzo beans, drained and rinsed

4 ounces feta cheese, crumbled

¾ cup basil, chopped

A pinch of salt and black pepper

2 tablespoons lemon juice

½ teaspoon lemon zest, grated

½ cup olive oil

DIRECTIONS

In a salad bowl, combine the brown rice with the arugula, the beans, and the rest of the ingredients, toss, and serve cold for breakfast.

NUTRITION Calories 473, Fat 22g, Fiber 7g, Carbs 53g, Protein 13g

Olive and Milk Bread

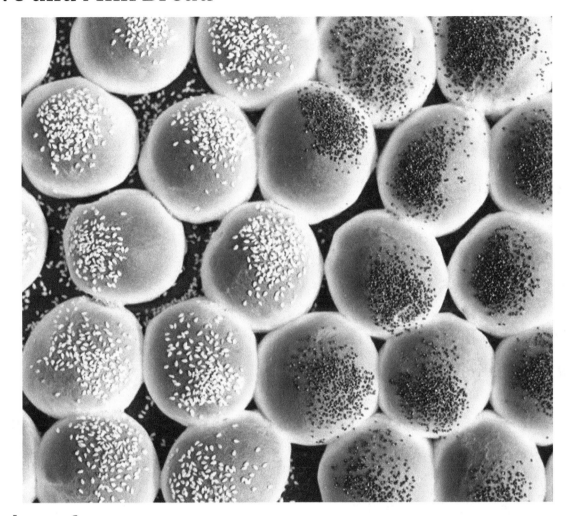

Servings: 6

Preparation time: 50 minutes

INGREDIENTS

- 1 cup black olives, pitted, chopped

- 1 tablespoon olive oil

- ½ teaspoon fresh yeast

- ½ cup milk, preheated

- ½ teaspoon salt

- 1 teaspoon baking powder

- 2 cup wheat flour, whole grain

- 2 eggs, beaten

- 1 teaspoon butter, melted

- 1 teaspoon sugar

DIRECTIONS

1. In the big bowl, combine together fresh yeast, sugar, and milk. Stir it until yeast is dissolved.

2. Then add salt, baking powder, butter, and eggs. Stir the dough mixture until homogenous and add 1 cup of wheat flour. Mix it up until smooth.

3. Add olives and remaining flour. Knead the non-sticky dough.

4. Transfer the dough into the non-sticky dough mold.

5. Bake the bread for 50 minutes at 350 F.

6. Check if the bread is cooked with the help of the toothpick. If it is dry, the bread is cooked.

7. Remove the bread from the oven and let it chill for 10-15 minutes.

8. Remove it from the loaf mold and slice.

NUTRITION Calories 238, Fat 7.7g, Fiber 1.9, Carbs 35.5g, Protein 7.2g

Blueberry and Vanilla Scones

Servings: 12

Preparation time: 20 minutes

INGREDIENTS

½ cup almond flour

3 manic eggs, beaten

2 tsp baking powder

½ cup stevia

2 tsp vanilla extract, unsweetened

¾ cup fresh raspberries

1 tbsp olive oil

DIRECTIONS

Switch on the oven, then set its temperature to 375 °F and let it preheat.

Take a large bowl, add flour and eggs in it, stir in baking powder, stevia, and vanilla until combined, and then fold in berries until mixed.

Take a baking dish, grease it with oil, scoop the prepared batter on it with an ice cream scoop and bake for 10 minutes until done.

When done, transfer scones on a wire rack, cool them completely, and then serve.

NUTRITION Calories 133, Total Fat 8g, Total Carbs 4g. Protein 2g

Tahini Pine Nuts Toast

Servings: 2

Preparation time: 0 minutes

INGREDIENTS

- 2 whole-wheat bread slices, toasted

- 1 teaspoon water

- 1 tablespoon tahini paste

- 2 teaspoons feta cheese, crumbled

- Juice of ½ lemon

- 2 teaspoons pine nuts

- A pinch of black pepper

DIRECTIONS

In a bowl, mix the tahini with the water and the lemon juice, whisk really well, and spread over the toasted bread slices.

Top each serving with the remaining ingredients and serve for breakfast.

NUTRITION Calories 142, Fat 7.6g, Fiber 2.7g, Carbs 13.7g, Protein 5.8g

Chili Scramble

Servings: 4

Preparation time: 15 minutes

INGREDIENTS

3 tomatoes

4 eggs

¼ teaspoon of sea salt

½ chili pepper, chopped

1 tablespoon butter

1 cup water for cooking

DIRECTIONS

Pour water into the saucepan and bring it to a boil.

Then remove water from the heat and add tomatoes.

Let the tomatoes stay in hot water for 2-3 minutes.

Then, remove the tomatoes from the water and peel them.

Place butter in the pan and melt it.

Add chopped chili pepper and fry it for 3 minutes over medium heat.

Then chop the peeled tomatoes and add them into the chili peppers.

Cook the vegetables for 5 minutes over medium heat. Stir them from time to time.

Then, add sea salt and crack then eggs.

Stir (scramble) the eggs well with the help of the fork and cook them for 3 minutes over medium heat.

NUTRITION Calories 105, Fat 7.4g, Fiber 1.1g, Carbs 4g, Protein 6.4g

Cheesy Caprese Style Portobellos Mushrooms

Servings: 2

Preparation time: 20 minutes

INGREDIENTS

2 large caps of Portobello mushroom, gills removed

4 tomatoes, halved

Salt and freshly cracked black pepper to taste

¼ cup fresh basil

4 tbsp olive oil

¼ cup shredded Mozzarella cheese

INSTRUCTIONS

1. Switch on the oven, then set its temperature to 400°F and let it preheat.

2. Place tomatoes in a bowl, season with salt and black pepper, add basil, drizzle with oil and toss until mixed.

3. Distribute cheese evenly in the bottom of each mushroom cap and then top with prepared tomato mixture.

4. Take a baking sheet, line it with aluminum foil, place prepared mushrooms on it and bake for some minutes until thoroughly cooked.

5. Serve straight away.

   NUTRITION Calories 315, Total Fat 29.2g, Total Carbs 14.2g, Protein 4.7g, Sugar 10.4g, Sodium 55mg

Pear Oatmeal

Servings: 4

Preparation time: 25 minutes

INGREDIENTS

1 cup oatmeal

1/3 cup milk

1 pear, chopped

1 teaspoon vanilla extract

1 tablespoon Splenda

1 teaspoon butter

½ teaspoon ground cinnamon

1 egg, beaten

DIRECTIONS

1. In the big bowl, mix up together oatmeal, milk, egg, vanilla extract, Splenda, and ground cinnamon.

2. Melt butter and add it to the oatmeal mixture.

3. Then add chopped pear and stir it well.

4. Transfer the oatmeal mixture to the casserole mold and flatten gently. Cover it with foil and secure edges.

5. Bake the oatmeal for 25 minutes at 350F.

NUTRITION Calories 151, Fat 3.9g, Fiber 3.3g, Carbs 23.6g, Protein 4.9g

Mediterranean Frittata

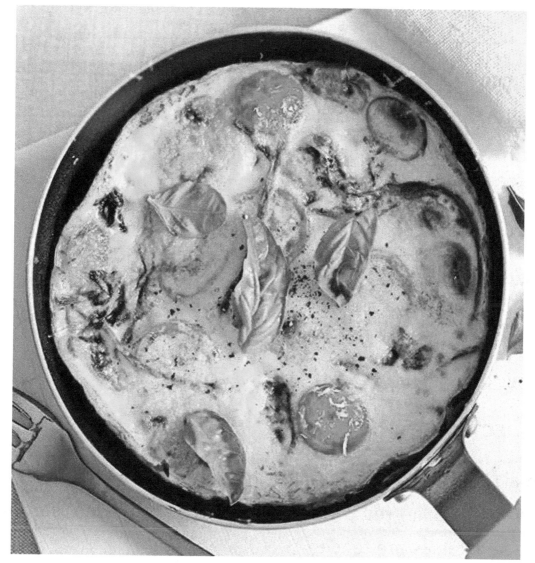

Servings: 6

Preparation time: 15 minutes

INGREDIENTS

- 9 large eggs, lightly beaten

- 8 kalamata olives, pitted, chopped

- ¼ cup olive oil

- 1/3 cup parmesan cheese, freshly grated

- 1/3 cup fresh basil, thinly sliced

- ½ teaspoon salt

- ½ teaspoon pepper

- ½ cup onion, chopped

- 1 sweet red pepper, diced

- 1 medium zucchini, cut to 1/2-inch cubes

- 1 package (4 ounces) feta cheese, crumbled

DIRECTIONS

1. In a 10-inch oven-proof skillet, heat the olive oil until hot. Add the olives, zucchini, red pepper, and onions, constantly stirring, until the vegetables are tender.

2. In a bowl, mix the eggs, feta cheese, basil, salt, and pepper; pour in the skillet with vegetables. Adjust heat to medium-low, cover, and cook for some minutes, or until the egg mixture is almost set.

3. Remove from the heat and sprinkle with the parmesan cheese. Transfer to the broiler.

4. With the oven door partially open, broil 5 ½ from the source of heat for about 2-3 minutes or until the top is golden. Cut into wedges.

NUTRITIONAL Calories 288.5, Fat 22.8g, Chol 301mg, Sodium 656 mg, Carb 5.6g, Fiber 1.2g, Sugar 3.3g, Protein 15.2g

Mediterranean Egg Casserole

Servings: 8

Preparation time: 50 minutes

INGREDIENTS

- 1 ½ cups (6 ounces) feta cheese, crumbled

- 1 jar (6 ounces) marinated artichoke hearts, drained well, coarsely chopped

- 10 eggs

- 2 cups milk, low-fat

- 2 cups fresh baby spinach, packed, coarsely chopped

- 6 cups whole-wheat baguette, cut into i-inch cubes

- 1 tablespoon garlic (about 4 cloves), finely chopped

- 1 tablespoon olive oil, extra-virgin

- ½ cup red bell pepper, chopped

- ½ cup Parmesan cheese, shredded

- ½ teaspoon pepper

- ½ teaspoon red pepper flakes

- ½ teaspoon salt

- 1/3 cup kalamata olives, pitted, halved

- ¼ cup red onion, chopped

- ¼ cup tomatoes (sun-dried) in oil, drained, chopped

DIRECTIONS

1. Preheat oven to 350 F.

2. Grease a 9x13 inch baking dish with olive oil cooking spray.

3. In an 8-inch non-stick pan over medium heat, heat the olive oil. Add the onions, garlic, and bell pepper; cook for about 3 minutes, frequently stirring, until slightly softened. Add the spinach; cook for about 1 minute or until starting to wilt.

4. Layer half of the baguette cubes in the prepared baking dish, then 1 cup of the feta, 1/4 cup Parmesan, the bell pepper mix, artichokes, the olives, and the tomatoes. Top with the remaining baguette cubes and then with the remaining ½ cup of feta.

5. In a large mixing bowl, whisk the eggs and the low-fat milk together. Beat in the pepper, salt, and pepper. Pour the mix over the bread layer in the baking dish, slightly pressing down. Sprinkle with the remaining ¼ cup Parmesan.

6. Bake for about 40-45 minutes, or until the center is set and the top is golden brown. Before serving, let stand for 15 minutes.

NUTRITION Calories 360, Fat 21g, Chol 270mg, Sodium 880mg, Carb 24g, Fiber 3g, Sugar 7g, Protein 20g

Egg Casserole with Paprika

Servings: 4

Preparation time: 40 minutes

INGREDIENTS

- 2 eggs, beaten

- 1 red bell pepper, chopped

- 1 chili pepper, chopped

- ½ red onion, diced

- 1 teaspoon canola oil

- ½ teaspoon salt

- 1 teaspoon paprika

- 1 tablespoon fresh cilantro, chopped

- 1 garlic clove, diced

- 1 teaspoon butter, softened

- ¼ teaspoon chili flakes

DIRECTIONS

Brush the casserole mold with canola oil and pour beaten eggs inside.

After this, toss the butter in the skillet and melt it over medium heat.

Add chili pepper and red bell pepper.

After this, add red onion and cook the vegetables for 7-8 minutes over medium heat. Stir them from time to time.

Transfer the vegetables to the casserole mold.

Add salt, paprika, cilantro, diced garlic, and chili flakes. Stir gently with the help of a spatula to get a homogenous mixture.

Bake the casserole for no minutes at 355F in the oven.

Then chill the meal well and cut into servings. Transfer the casserole to the serving plates with the help of the spatula.

NUTRITION: Calories 168, Fat 12,3, Fiber 1.5g, Carbs 4 4g, Protein 8.8g

Paprika Salmon Toast

Servings: 2

Preparation time: 3 minutes

INGREDIENTS

- 4 whole-grain bread slices

- 2 oz smoked salmon, sliced

- 2 teaspoons cream cheese

- 1 teaspoon fresh dill, chopped

- ½ teaspoon lemon juice

- ½ teaspoon paprika

- 4 lettuce leaves

- 1 cucumber, sliced

DIRECTIONS

Toast the bread in the toaster (1-2 minutes totally).

In the bowl, mix up together fresh dill, cream cheese, lemon juice, and paprika.

Then spread the toasts with the cream cheese mixture.

Slice the smoked salmon and place it on bread slices.

Add sliced cucumber and lettuce leaves.

Top the lettuce with remaining bread toasts and pin with the toothpick.

NUTRITION Calories 202, Fat 4.7g, Fiber 5.1g, Carbs 31.5g, Protein 12.7g

Scrambled Eggs

Servings: 2

Preparation time: 10 minutes

INGREDIENTS

- 1 yellow bell pepper, chopped

- 8 cherry tomatoes, cubed

- 2 spring onions, chopped

- 1 tablespoon olive oil

- 1 tablespoon capers, drained

- 2 tablespoons black olives, pitted and sliced

- 4 eggs

- A pinch of salt and black pepper

- ¼ teaspoon oregano, dried

- 1 tablespoon parsley, chopped

DIRECTIONS

1. Heat up a pan with the oil over medium-high heat, add the bell pepper and spring onions and sauté for 3 minutes.

2. Add the tomatoes, capers, and olives and sauté for a minute.

3. Crack the eggs into the pan, add salt, pepper, oregano, and scramble for 5 minutes more.

4. Divide the scramble between plates, sprinkle the parsley on top, and serve.

NUTRITION Calories 249, Fat 17g, Fiber 3.2g, Carbs 13.3g, Protein 13.5g

Cheesy Olives Bread

Servings: 10

Preparation time: 30 minutes

INGREDIENTS

4 cups whole-wheat flour

3 tablespoons oregano, chopped

2 teaspoons dry yeast

¼ cup olive oil

1 and ½ cups black olives, pitted and sliced

1 cup water

½ cup feta cheese, crumbled

DIRECTIONS

1. In a bowl, mix the flour with the water, the yeast, and the oil, stir, and knead your dough very well.

2. Put the dough in a bowl, cover with plastic wrap and keep in a warm place for 1 hour.

3. Divide the dough into 2 bowls and stretch each ball really well.

4. Add the rest of the ingredients on each ball and tuck them inside, well kneading the dough again.

5. Flatten the balls a bit and leave them aside for 4 minutes more.

6. Transfer the balls to a baking sheet lined with parchment paper, make a small slit in each, and bake at 425 degrees F for 30 minutes.

7. Serve the bread as a Mediterranean breakfast.

NUTRITION Calories 251, Fat 7.3g, Fiber 2.1g, Carbs 39.7g, Protein 6.7g

Mediterranean Freezer Breakfast Wraps

Servings: 4

Preparation time: 3 minutes

INGREDIENTS

1 cup spinach leaves, fresh, chopped

1 tablespoon water or low-fat milk

½ teaspoon garlic-chipotle seasoning or your preferred seasoning

4 eggs, beaten

4 pieces (8-inch) whole-wheat tortillas

4 tablespoons tomato chutney (or dried tomatoes, chopped or calmed tomatoes)

4 tablespoons feta cheese, crumbled (or goat cheese)

Optional: prosciutto, chopped or bacon, cooked, crumbled

Salt and pepper to taste

DIRECTIONS

1. In a mixing bowl, whisk the eggs, water, or milk, and seasoning together.

2. Heat a skillet with a little olive oil; pour the eggs and scramble for about 3-4 minutes, or until just cooked.

3. Lay the tortillas on a clean surface; divide the eggs between them, arranging the scrambled eggs, and leave the tortilla edges free to fold later.

4. Top the egg layer with about 1 tablespoon of cheese, 1 tablespoon of tomatoes, and 1/ 4 cup spinach. If using, layer with prosciutto or bacon.

5. In a burrito-style, roll up the tortillas, folding both of the ends in the process.

6. In a panini maker or a clean skillet, cook for about 1 minute, turning once, until the tortilla wraps are crisp and brown; serve.

NUTRITION Calories 450, Fat 15g, Chol 220mg, Sodium 280mg, Pot. 960mg, Carb 64g, Fiber 6g, Sugar 20g, Protein 17g

Milk Scones

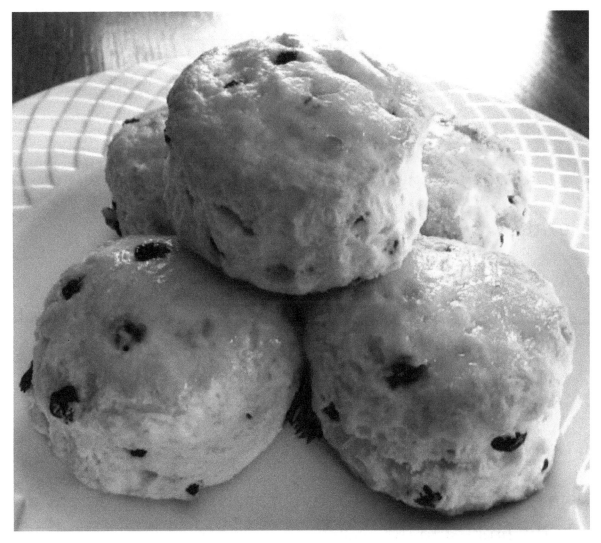

Servings: 4

Preparation time: 10 minutes

INGREDIENTS

- ½ cup wheat flour, whole grain

- 1 teaspoon baking powder

- 1 tablespoon butter, melted

- 1 teaspoon vanilla extract

- 1 egg, beaten

- ¾ teaspoon salt

- 3 tablespoons milk

- 1 teaspoon vanilla sugar

DIRECTIONS

1. In the mixing bowl, combine together wheat flour, baking powder, butter, vanilla extract, and egg. Add salt and knead the soft and non-sticky dough. Add more flour if needed.

2. Then make the log from the dough and cut it into triangles.

3. Line the tray with baking paper.

4. Arrange the dough triangles on the baking paper and transfer them to the preheat to the 360F oven.

5. Cook the scones for 10 minutes or until they are light brown.

6. Then chill the scones and brush with milk and sprinkle with vanilla sugar.

   NUTRITION Calories 112, Fat 4.4g, Fiber 0.5g, Carbs 14.3g, Protein 3.4g

Herbed Eggs and Mushroom Mix

Servings: 4

Preparation time: 20 minutes

INGREDIENTS

- 1 red onion, chopped

- 1 bell pepper, chopped

- 1 tablespoon tomato paste

- 1/3 cup water

- ½ teaspoon of sea salt

- 1 tablespoon butter

- 1 cup cremini mushrooms, chopped

- 1 tablespoon fresh parsley

- 1 tablespoon fresh dill

- 1 teaspoon dried thyme

- ½ teaspoon dried oregano

- ½ teaspoon paprika

- ½ teaspoon chili flakes

- ½ teaspoon garlic powder

- 4 eggs

DIRECTIONS

1. Toss butter in the pan and melt it.

2. Then add chopped mushrooms and bell pepper.

3. Roast the vegetables for 5 minutes over medium heat.

4. Then add onion and stir well.

5. Sprinkle the ingredients with garlic powder, chili flakes, dried oregano, and dried thyme. Mix up well

6. Then add tomato paste and water.

7. Mix up the mixture until it is homogenous.

8. Then add fresh parsley and dill.

9. Cook the mixture for 5 minutes over medium-high heat with the closed lid.

10. After this, stir the mixture with the help of the spatula well.

11. Crack the eggs over the mixture and close the lid.

12. Cook for 10 minutes over low heat.

NUTRITION Calories 123, Fat 7.5g, Fiber 1.7g, Carbs 7.8, Protein 7.1g

Leeks and Eggs Muffins

Servings: 2

Preparation time: 20 minutes

INGREDIENTS

3 eggs, whisked

¼ cup baby spinach

2 tablespoons leeks, chopped

4 tablespoons parmesan, grated

2 tablespoons almond milk

Cooking spray

1 small red bell pepper, chopped

Salt and black pepper to the taste

1 tomato, cubed

2 tablespoons cheddar cheese, grated

DIRECTIONS

1. In a bowl, combine the eggs with the milk, salt, pepper, and the rest of the ingredients except the cooking spray and whisk well.

2. Grease a muffin tin with the cooking spray and divide the egg mixture in each muffin mould.

3. Bake at 380 degrees F for no minutes and serve them for breakfast.

   NUTRITION Calories 308, Fat 19.4g, Fiber 1.7g, Carbs 8.7g, Protein 24.4g

Mango and Spinach Bowls

Servings: 4

Preparation time: 0 minutes

INGREDIENTS

- 1 cup baby arugula

- 1 cup baby spinach, chopped

- 1 mango, peeled and cubed

- 1 cup strawberries, halved

- 1 tablespoon hemp seeds

- 1 cucumber, sliced

- 1 tablespoon lime juice

- 1 tablespoon tahini paste

- 1 tablespoon water

DIRECTIONS

In a salad bowl, mix the arugula with the rest of the ingredients except the tahini and the water and toss.

In a small bowl, combine the tahini with the water, whisk well, add to the salad, toss, divide into small bowls and serve for breakfast.

NUTRITION Calories 211, Fat 4.5g, Fiber 6.5g, Carbs 10.2g, Protein 3.5g

Figs Oatmeal

Servings: 5

Preparation time: 20 minutes

INGREDIENTS

- 2 cups oatmeal

- 1 ½ cup milk

- 1 tablespoon butter

- 3 figs, chopped

- 1 tablespoon honey

DIRECTIONS

1. Pour milk into the saucepan.

2. Add oatmeal and close the lid.

3. Cook the oatmeal for 15 minutes over medium-low heat.

4. Then add chopped figs and honey.

5. Add butter and mix up the oatmeal well.

6. Cook it for 5 minutes more.

7. Close the lid and let the cooked breakfast rest for 10 minutes before serving.

NUTRITION Calories 222, Fat 6, Fiber 4.4g, carbs 36.5g, Protein 7.1g

Veggie Quiche

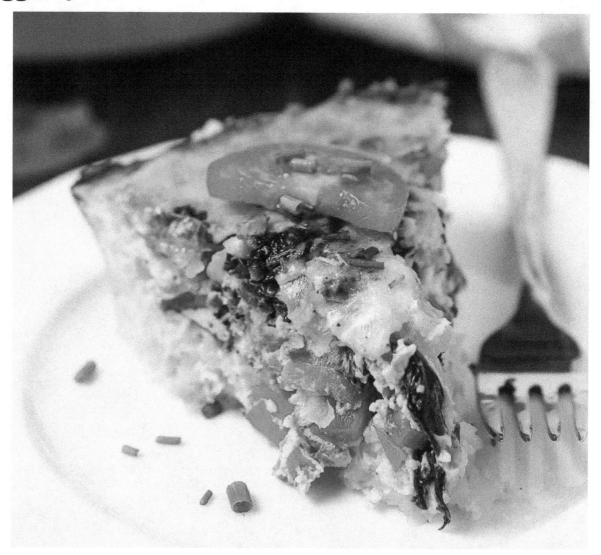

Servings: 8

Preparation time: 55 minutes

INGREDIENTS

½ cup sun-dried tomatoes, chopped

1 prepared pie crust

2 tablespoons avocado oil

1 yellow onion, chopped

2 garlic cloves, minced

2 cups spinach, chopped

1 red bell pepper, chopped

¼ cup kalamata olives, pitted and sliced

1 teaspoon parsley flakes

1 teaspoon oregano, dried

1/3 cup feta cheese, crumbled

4 eggs, whisked

1 and ½ cups almond milk

1 cup cheddar cheese, shredded

Salt and black pepper to the taste

DIRECTIONS

1. Heat up a pan with the oil over medium-high heat, add the garlic and onion and sauté for 3 minutes.

2. Add the bell pepper and sauté for 3 minutes more.

3. Add the olives, parsley, spinach, oregano, salt, pepper, and cook everything for some minutes.

4. Add tomatoes and the cheese, toss and take off the heat.

5. Arrange the pie crust on a pie plate, pour the spinach and tomatoes mix inside and spread.

6. In a bowl, mix the eggs with salt, pepper, milk, and half of the cheese, whisk and pour over the mixture in the pie crust.

7. Sprinkle the remaining cheese on top and bake at 375 degrees F for 40 minutes.

8. Cool the quiche down, slice, and serve for breakfast.

NUTRITION Calories 211, Fat 14 4g, Fiber 1.4g, Carbs 12.5g, Protein 8.6g

Conclusion

I am so interested to see what delicious dishes you have actually produced.

I make certain you've been hectic and we've delighted the palates of friends and family.

Do not stop working out and maintain trying these recipes. They are distinct, healthy as well as nourishing. Perfect for the whole family members.

I constantly recommend talking to a nutritionist before any kind of nutritional modifications, and getting a lot of physical activity.

I thanks and eagerly anticipate future dishes.

CPSIA information can be obtained
at www.ICGtesting.com
Printed in the USA
LVHW061221110521
687091LV00008B/1459